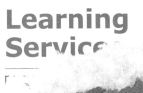

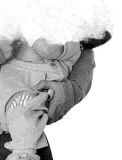

baby
first aid
Dr. **miriam**
stoppard

A Dorling Kindersley Book

LONDON, NEW YORK,
MELBOURNE AND DELHI

Design: Nick Harris
Editor: Jinny Johnson

Category Publisher:
Corinne Roberts

Senior Managing Art Editor:
Lynne Brown

Art Editor:
Rosamund Saunders

Senior Editor:
Peter Jones

Designer:
Carla de Abreu

Consultant:
Jemima Dunne

Production Controller:
Heather Hughes

DTP Designer:
Karen Constanti

For Olivia

First published in Great Britain in 2003 by
Dorling Kindersley Limited,
80 Strand, London WC2R ORL

A Penguin Company

A CIP catalogue record for this book is
available from the British Library.

ISBN 1405 301 430

Reproduced by GRB, Italy
Printed by TBB, Slovakia

See our complete catalogue at
www.dk.com

contents

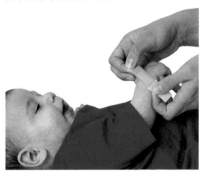

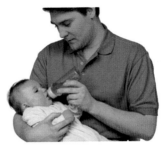

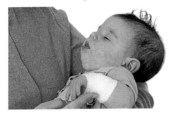

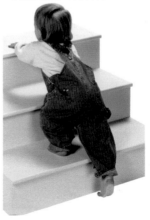

Introduction

When your child suddenly needs urgent medical attention it's hard to stay calm and decisive. But you're no good to your child if you panic. The best way to control your surging anxiety is to take several slow deep breaths and reach for this book.

Here I've tried to lay out a simple step-by-step action plan for you to follow when faced with the most common medical emergencies, from deep cuts and burns to accidents that are in themselves minor, but nonetheless upset your child, like splinters and blisters.

The advice given in this book applies to boys and girls alike so I have simply alternated "he" and "she" throughout.

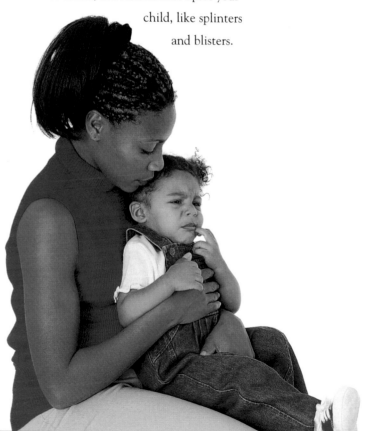

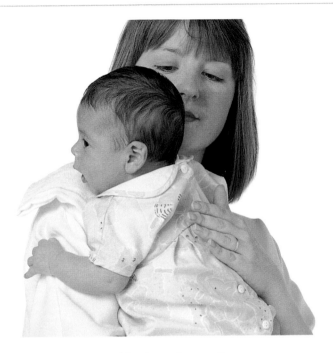

This is a BABY first aid book so it's specially tailored for parents of children under three.

It's quite a good idea to read the book through so that you're prearmed in the event that an emergency should strike your family.

The remedies and techniques I suggest recognize the sometimes frighteningly tiny size of babies and I hope that will encourage you to act with confidence and expediency.

It can be dangerous to perform some of the emergency procedures on babies unless absolutely necessary. You can do serious harm so never rehearse these actions. Because of this, the photographs show dummies, not real babies, to illustrate these points.

HOME FIRST AID

All parents have to deal with minor accidents from time to time, especially after babies learn to walk and get more adventurous. It's a good idea to keep a first-aid kit at home and in the car, and a more extensive medicine chest at home as well. Check supplies regularly to make sure you haven't run out of anything. And keep medicines and first-aid kits well out of children's reach.

first-aid supplies

Keep these items in a clearly marked box with an airtight lid. Make sure you know how to use each one properly.

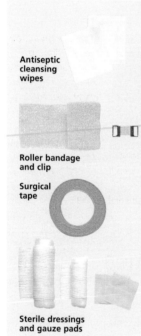

Antiseptic cleansing wipes

Roller bandage and clip

Surgical tape

Sterile dressings and gauze pads

- **Box of assorted adhesive dressings**, or plasters. Children love colourful plasters, but keep some of the hypoallergenic type as well, because some people are allergic to the adhesive used in standard plasters
- **2–3 roller bandages** for securing dressings. Keep several different sizes and some clips or safety pins
- **Crepe or conforming bandages** are useful for supporting sprains and strains. Keep at least one
- **2–3 sterile wound dressings** These are pads that have bandages attached, ideal for larger wounds
- **Sterile non-adhesive dressings** with a shiny coating on one side that's easy to peel off a wound. The dressings need to be secured with a bandage or tape
- **Surgical tape** for holding dressings in place
- **1–2 triangular bandages** These can be used to make a sling or for covering a wound
- **Finger bandage and applicator** This is quick and easy to apply to a finger or toe injury
- **Antiseptic cleansing wipes** for cleaning wounds. Make sure they are alcohol free
- **Pack of gauze pads** for cleaning around a wound or as extra padding when dealing with bleeding

useful equipment

- **Blunt-ended scissors**
- **Tweezers**
- **Disposable gloves**
- **Emergency face mask** for resuscitation
- **Torch** in the event of electricity failing

USEFUL EQUIPMENT FOR THE CAR
- **First-aid kit**
- **Foil emergency blanket and a torch**
- **Whistle** for attracting attention
- **Spare nappy changing kit**

home medicine chest

With medicines or ointments, always read the label and follow instructions carefully. Some may not be recommended for use in very young children.

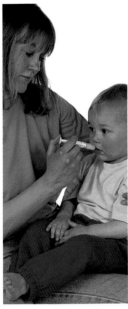

Using a 5ml oral syringe

- **Junior ibuprofen** and/or infant paracetamol for treating pain or fever in babies and young children. Don't give these to babies under three months unless your doctor recommends it. In severe cases these medications can be used together
- **5ml oral syringe** for giving medicines to babies and young children
- **Calamine lotion** or cream for soothing skin irritation or sunburn
- **Emollient cream and bath oil** for dry skin
- **Sachets of rehydration salts** When mixed with water these can be given to babies and young children to replace salts lost by severe vomiting and diarrhoea and to prevent dehydration
- **Sunblock cream** Replace your supplies at least every summer
- **Thermometer** Use a feverscan thermometer that can be put on your baby's head, or a digital read-out thermometer under the armpit. A more expensive but very effective option is an aural thermometer (used in the ear). It takes only a few seconds to get a reading and can be used when your child is asleep

complementary remedies

I know how keen some parents are to use natural and herbal remedies themselves and would also consider giving them to their children. So that I could give you sound and safe medical advice, I undertook some research on these remedies on your behalf.

I cannot recommend the following complementary and alternative remedies commonly suggested for use in children:

- **Chamomilla**, for teething, can trigger allergies and anaphylactic shock
- **Cocculus**, for travel sickness, can cause kidney failure
- **Nux vomica**, for colic, can contain strychnine

In fact, only two remedies are safe for babies:

- **Arnica cream** supposedly for bruises
- **Calendula cream** for abrasions

But these two are **not** effective. In fact, a recent study has shown arnica to be totally ineffective for bruising and swelling.

USING DRESSINGS AND BANDAGES

Covering a wound with a clean, dry dressing will help prevent the area becoming infected as well as help to stop any bleeding. Putting a plaster or dressing on a wound will also reassure your child – children are often very frightened by the sight of blood, especially their own. Whether you use a plaster or a wound dressing, always make sure that the pad is larger than the wound. If you put a bandage around a limb, always check the blood circulation in the limb beyond the bandage to make sure it's not too tight.

putting on a plaster

Remove the outer wrapper, then hold the plaster, dressing side down, over the wound. Peel back the protective layer, and place the dressing on the wound. Press down the ends and edges of the plaster securely.

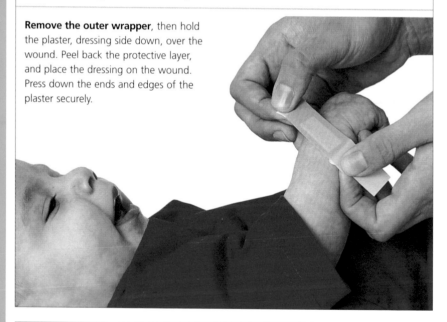

putting on a wound dressing

1 **Put on disposable gloves** if you have them, then remove the dressing's outer wrapper. Unroll the bandage to open up the dressing pad, making sure that you don't touch it.

2 **Place the dressing pad** on the wound and wind the short end of the bandage once around the pad to secure it, then leave it hanging. Wrap the main bandage around the limb until the pad is completely covered. Then tie both ends of the bandage in a knot over the pad to keep pressure on the wound.

putting on a roller bandage

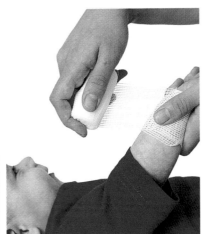

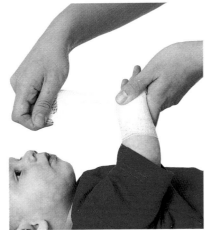

1 **Support the injured limb** with your hand. Unroll part of the bandage and place it on the limb below the injury, keeping the rolled-up section uppermost.

2 **Wind the bandage** around the limb working up the limb, so that each layer of bandage covers about two-thirds of the previous layer. When the dressing or injury is completely covered, finish off with two straight turns, then secure the end with a safety pin, bandage clip or adhesive tape.

CHECKING CIRCULATION AFTER BANDAGING

Press on your child's fingernail or toenail beyond the bandage, then release the pressure. The normal colour of the nail should come back quickly. If the colour doesn't return, the bandage is too tight. Undo the bandage, wait for the colour to return to normal, and put the bandage on again more loosely.

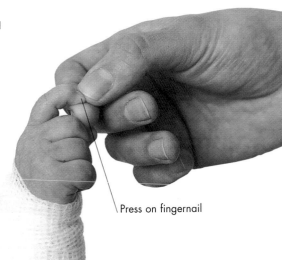

Press on fingernail

WHAT TO DO IN THE EVENT OF AN INCIDENT

It can be very distressing for parents when their baby or toddler is ill or injured. It isn't always easy for a parent to know what to do immediately and it may be unclear whether an injury is serious, or even potentially serious. Whatever happens, if you're in any doubt, follow your instincts. If you're worried, call your doctor for advice.

immediate action

In the event of an incident, stay calm. Make sure the area around your child is safe. If you injure yourself in the process of rescuing or helping your child, you'll put her in greater danger. Reassure your child. Call the relevant emergency service – ambulance, police, or fire service.

1 **Make sure the area** around your child is safe for you to approach her. For example, if your child is in contact with electricity, turn off the electricity supply before you touch her.

2 **Assess your child** to make sure she's conscious and breathing (baby p.16; child p.19). If she's conscious, go to step 3.

3 **Assess any injuries**. If your child is conscious assess her injuries and treat as necessary. Call your doctor for advice or ring for an ambulance, see opposite.

WARNING

- If your child is unconscious, follow the procedure for an unconscious baby p.16 or toddler p.19. Check your child's breathing, then ask someone to call an ambulance while you continue treating her.
- If your child isn't breathing and you're on your own, give rescue breaths and chest compressions for a minute, then call an ambulance.
- Unconsciousness takes precedence over all other injuries – including bleeding.

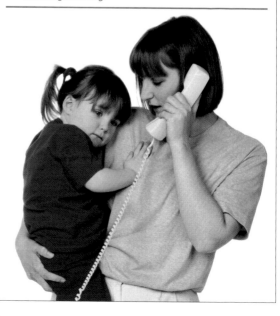

SEE ALSO

- *If it's necessary to call an ambulance, monitor your child's condition carefully while waiting for help to arrive (see Monitoring vital signs p.12)*

when to get a child to hospital

These situations are all serious enough to require admission to hospital. Many are real emergencies, in which case you should call an ambulance. Ambulance personnel are highly skilled in first aid and well equipped, but knowing what to do before they arrive could save your child's life. Specific advice about each of the situations mentioned here is given elsewhere in this book.

ALWAYS GET YOUR BABY OR YOUNG CHILD TO HOSPITAL IF SHE HAS:
- **lost consciousness**
- **stopped breathing**
- **difficulty breathing**
- **sustained a deep wound**, or a wound with an embedded object
- **any burn**
- **a raised temperature** accompanied by drowsiness and a purplish rash on the body, sensitivity to light, headache, and/or stiff neck (see meningitis p.56)
- **a head injury**
- **a suspected broken bone**
- **eaten a poisonous substance** (for example berries, medicine, or chemicals)
- **a chemical burn** on skin or in her eyes
- **a foreign object** lodged in her ear, nose or eye
- **a snake or animal bite, or insect bite** if there's a family history of severe allergic reactions

when to call a doctor

Most doctors won't mind if you consult them for advice. You know better than anyone whether your child is ill or not, and doctors ignore your opinion at their peril. So if in doubt, check with your doctor, especially if any of these important signs of illness is noted. If you cannot contact your doctor, take your child to your nearest accident and emergency department.

ALWAYS CALL YOUR DOCTOR FOR ADVICE IN THE FOLLOWING SITUATIONS:
- **If a baby or child has a raised temperature** of 39°C (102.2°F) or more, or if your child has had a fever of over 38°C (100.4°F) for more than three days
- **Raised temperature accompanied by seizures** or if your child has had seizures with fevers in the past
- **Raised temperature that has dropped then rises** again suddenly
- **Body temperature below 35°C (95°F)** accompanied by cold skin, drowsiness, quietness, and listlessness (see hypothermia p.50)
- **If a baby has been vomiting** for more than six hours
- **If a baby or child has prolonged violent vomiting**
- **If a child complains of dizzy spells** plus nausea and headaches, or nausea and vomiting accompanied by right-sided abdominal pain
- **If a baby goes off her food suddenly**, or a child who usually has a healthy appetite refuses food for a day and seems listless

MONITORING VITAL SIGNS

If you think your child is ill and in need of medical attention, check his vital signs – level of response, breathing rate, and pulse. The more information you give your doctors when you call, the better they'll be able to help you.

checking level of response

To find out whether your child is conscious and to monitor any change in his condition, you need to check his level of response to certain stimuli at regular intervals. Write down the results and the time of the assessments and give them to the doctor or ambulance personnel.

1 Talk to your child – is he alert, does he open his eyes and maintain normal eye contact with you?

2 Does your child respond to your voice? For example, does he turn his head towards you (baby), respond sensibly to questioning (toddler), or does he seem very confused? Or is there no response?

3 Is he moving? Tap his foot (baby) or his shoulder (toddler) and see if he reacts. If there's no reaction, he may have lost consciousness. Go to pp.14–21 for guidelines on resuscitation techniques.

checking breathing rates

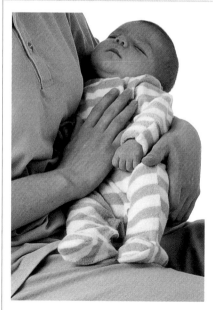

Rapid or very slow breathing or difficulty in breathing can be a sign that a child needs urgent medical help. To check your child's breathing rate, keep him still and count the number of breaths he takes in a minute. Normal rates per minute are as follows:

BREATHS PER MINUTE:

Under 2 months: 50–60 breaths or less
2–12 months: 40–50 breaths or less
1–2 years: 30 breaths or less

WARNING

• Difficulty in breathing is a medical emergency and a sign that a child needs immediate help. If your child's lips go blue, send for an ambulance immediately.

checking your child's pulse

A rapid or very slow pulse is another sign that your child is unwell. Note, too, whether the pulse is strong or weak. Average pulse rates are as follows:

BEATS PER MINUTE:
Under 2 months: 100–160
Over 1: 100–120

Using your first two fingers, count the beats for 15 seconds and multiply by four.

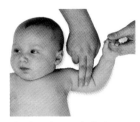

check pulse on baby's arm   **check pulse on child's wrist**

taking your child's temperature

In children, normal body temperature ranges from 36°C (96.8°F) to 37°C (98.6°F). Any temperature over 37.7°C (100°F) is classed as a fever. A hot forehead may be the first sign that your child has a temperature, but to be accurate, you must take your child's temperature with a thermometer, and then take it again after 20 minutes.

TIPS FOR TAKING YOUR CHILD'S TEMPERATURE

- **Always read** the manufacturer's instructions carefully.
- **Never take your child's temperature** if he has just stopped running about.
- **Wash the thermometer** after use with soap and cold water.
- **Always store** the thermometer in its own case.

DIFFERENT TYPES OF THERMOMETERS

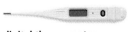

digital thermometer

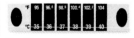

liquid crystal strip

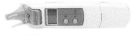

aural thermometer

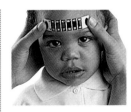

Hold the strip against your child's forehead with both hands, keeping your fingers clear of the panels. Make sure the strip is flat against your child's forehead.

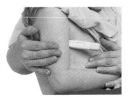

Put a digital thermometer into the armpit and lower your child's arm over it. Hold the arm down until the thermometer bleeps, then remove and read it.

UNCONSCIOUS BABIES AND TODDLERS

If a baby or toddler has lost consciousness and isn't breathing, she's at risk of brain damage and cardiac arrest. Resuscitation is vital – getting oxygen into your child's lungs and making sure her heart is beating. You need to make a fast assessment of your child's condition in order to know what to do. The plan of action opposite will help. An easy way to remember what to do is to follow the ABC of resuscitation (below).

Note that resuscitation techniques are slightly different for babies under 12 months and for toddlers, as the following pages will show.

ABC of resuscitation

A = airway

A= Airway, which must be kept open and clear. If a baby or child becomes unconscious and is lying on her back, there is a danger that her tongue will fall back, blocking the airway so that air containing oxygen cannot enter the lungs. By tilting her head back, you may be able to open the airway enough to enable breathing.

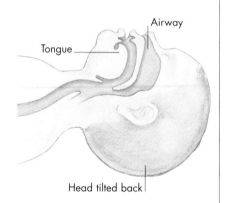

Airway

Tongue

Head tilted back

B = breathing

B = Breathing, which must be maintained by keeping the airway open. Or you can sustain breathing artificially with rescue breaths (baby p.17; toddler p.20). This is possible because the air you breathe out contains enough oxygen to keep another person alive.

C = circulation

C = Circulation, which is vital in order to keep blood containing oxygen supplying the body tissues. If necessary, circulation can be partially kept going by imitating the heart action using chest compressions. Combined with rescue breathing, this may be enough to keep a child's system supplied with oxygen until ambulance personnel can take over. This is known as **cardiopulmonary resuscitation** (CPR).

plan of action

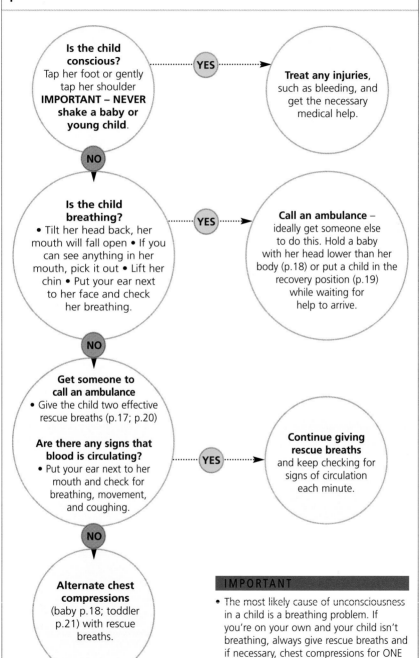

Is the child conscious?
Tap her foot or gently tap her shoulder **IMPORTANT – NEVER shake a baby or young child.**

···· **YES** ····▸

Treat any injuries, such as bleeding, and get the necessary medical help.

NO ▾

Is the child breathing?
• Tilt her head back, her mouth will fall open • If you can see anything in her mouth, pick it out • Lift her chin • Put your ear next to her face and check her breathing.

···· **YES** ····▸

Call an ambulance – ideally get someone else to do this. Hold a baby with her head lower than her body (p.18) or put a child in the recovery position (p.19) while waiting for help to arrive.

NO ▾

Get someone to call an ambulance
• Give the child two effective rescue breaths (p.17; p.20)

Are there any signs that blood is circulating?
• Put your ear next to her mouth and check for breathing, movement, and coughing.

···· **YES** ····▸

Continue giving rescue breaths and keep checking for signs of circulation each minute.

NO ▾

Alternate chest compressions (baby p.18; toddler p.21) with rescue breaths.

IMPORTANT

• The most likely cause of unconsciousness in a child is a breathing problem. If you're on your own and your child isn't breathing, always give rescue breaths and if necessary, chest compressions for ONE minute before you call an ambulance.

UNCONSCIOUS BABY

Follow the sequence of the next three pages to treat an unconscious baby of under 12 months. Always check he's breathing before calling an ambulance, as this is the first question the ambulance control officer will ask you. If possible, get someone else to make the call while you tend to the baby.

checking consciousness

If the baby has collapsed, you need to find out quickly whether or not he's conscious.

IMPORTANT
• Never shake a baby to check for response.

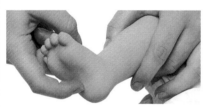

1 **Tap the sole of his foot** and call his name. This should be enough to get a response from him if he's asleep.

2 **If there is no reaction** at all, he's unconscious. If there's a reaction, treat any injury and call for help if necessary.

checking breathing

It's important to open a baby's airway before checking breathing because in an unconscious baby, the tongue will fall back across the top of the windpipe, preventing air from getting into the lungs.

IMPORTANT
• Never put your fingers into a baby's mouth to feel for an obstruction you cannot see.

1 **Put one hand on the baby's forehead,** and gently tilt the head back. Look in his mouth. If you can clearly see an obstruction pick it out with your finger and thumb.

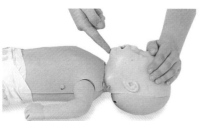

2 **Lift his chin with one finger** of your other hand to keep the airway open.

3 **Put your ear next to the baby's face** and look along his chest. Watch to see if his chest is moving, listen for breaths and feel for breaths on your cheek.

4 **If there are definite signs** of breathing, cradle the baby in your arms with his head lower than his body to keep the airway clear. Get someone to call an ambulance, or if necessary, take the baby to the telephone and call an ambulance yourself. Monitor the baby's vital signs (p.12) while waiting for help.

5 **If the baby is not breathing,** you must begin rescue breathing (opposite).

giving a baby rescue breaths

If the baby isn't breathing, you must get air into his body by blowing your exhaled air into his lungs. This works because your breath still has enough oxygen in it to keep another person alive. Get someone else to call for an ambulance. If you're on your own, continue rescue breathing for ONE minute before calling an ambulance, since the longer the baby's brain is starved of oxygen, the worse the consequences could be. Make sure you also know what to do if his heart stops beating (p.18).

1 Make sure his airway is open by supporting the head with both hands.

2 Take a deep breath, then seal your lips around the baby's mouth and nose. Blow steadily into the baby's lungs until you see the chest rise, then remove your mouth and watch the chest fall. This is called an effective breath.

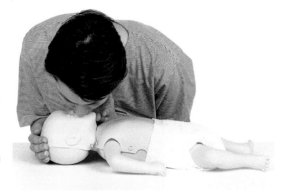

3 If the chest doesn't rise, reposition the baby's head to make sure the airway is open, check the mouth for obstructions, then try again. Try up to five times, stopping as soon as you manage to get two effective breaths into the baby's mouth.

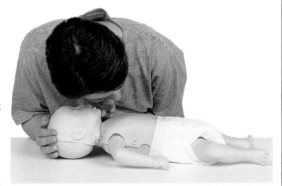

WARNING

- If you still cannot get the breaths in after five attempts, then go on to check the baby's circulation (step 4).
- If you cannot get the breaths in and you know the baby choked on something, don't check circulation, begin CPR (p.18) straightaway.

4 Check for signs of circulation. Put your ear close to the baby's face again and look for signs of movement, breathing or coughing for no more than 10 seconds. If you see signs, continue with rescue breaths for ONE minute – at a rate of about 20 breaths per minute – then repeat the circulation check. If the baby starts breathing, hold him in your arms while waiting for the ambulance.

5 Start CPR (cardiopulmonary resuscitation) if there are no signs of circulation. Follow the guidelines on p.18.

giving a baby CPR

CPR (cardiopulmonary resuscitation), involving chest compressions and rescue breaths, is necessary if the baby shows no signs of blood circulation. Through CPR it is possible to maintain some circulation. You should use only two fingers to give chest compressions for a baby.

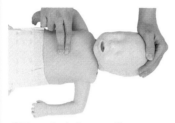
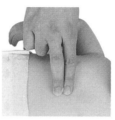
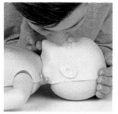

1 **Place the baby on a firm surface** (a table is ideal). Support her head with the hand nearest her head, and place the first two fingers of your other hand on the centre of the baby's chest (on the breastbone), about a finger's width below the baby's nipples.

2 **Press down sharply** on the breastbone to one third of its depth, then release the pressure (but don't remove your fingers). Do this five times at about 100 compressions per minute.

3 **Then give one rescue breath** into the baby's mouth and nose.

CONTINUE CHEST COMPRESSIONS AND RESCUE BREATHS

Continue giving five chest compressions followed by one rescue breath at this rate until the ambulance arrives, the baby starts moving or breathing, or you're too exhausted to keep going.

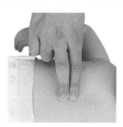
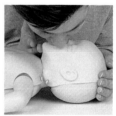

five compressions   **one rescue breath**

IF THE BABY STARTS TO BREATHE

Once the baby starts breathing on her own again and her circulation has returned, hold her in your arms, ideally face downwards, with her head lower than the main part of her body. This is known as the recovery position. The aims of the recovery position are:

• to keep the airway open
• to allow vomit and other fluids to drain from the mouth
• to keep the neck and spine aligned
While she is in the recovery position, keep monitoring her vital signs (p.12) carefully until an ambulance arrives.

UNCONSCIOUS TODDLER

Follow the sequence on the next few pages to treat an unconscious toddler over the age of 12 months. Always check her breathing before calling an ambulance, as this is the first question the ambulance control officer asks.

checking consciousness

When you find a collapsed toddler you need to find out immediately whether or not she is conscious. You must never shake a child.

1 **Gently tap her shoulder** and call her name, or you can blow gently on her eyelashes. This should be enough to get a response if she's asleep. Never shake her.

2 **If there is no reaction at all**, she is unconscious. Go to checking breathing (below). If there is a reaction, treat any injury and if necessary call for help.

checking breathing

It's important to open the airway before checking breathing. This is because in an unconscious toddler, her tongue will fall back across the top of the windpipe, preventing air from getting into her lungs.

1 **Put one hand on the child's forehead**, and gently tilt the head back (the mouth should fall open). Look in the child's mouth and if you can clearly see an obstruction, pick it out with your finger and thumb.

IMPORTANT

- Never put your fingers into a child's mouth to feel for an unseen obstruction – you might push it further down.

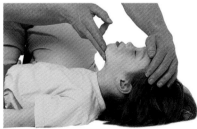

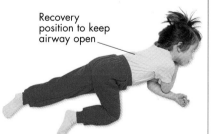

Recovery position to keep airway open

2 **Lift the child's chin** with two fingers of your other hand to keep the airway open.

3 **Put your ear next to the child's face** and look along her chest. Watch to see if her chest is moving, listen for breaths and feel for breaths on your cheek.

4 **If there are definite signs** of breathing, place your child on her side in the recovery position, with her head well back.

5 **If the child isn't breathing**, then you must begin rescue breathing (p.20).

giving a toddler rescue breaths

If the toddler isn't breathing, you must get air into her body by blowing your exhaled air into her lungs (rescue breathing). If you're on your own, you must try rescue breathing for ONE minute before calling an ambulance.

1 **Make sure her airway is open** by supporting the head with both hands. Pinch her nostrils together with one hand.

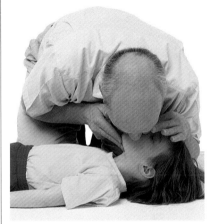 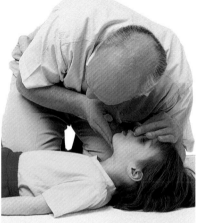

2 **Take a deep breath**, then seal your lips around the child's mouth and blow steadily into her lungs until you see her chest rise. Remove your mouth and watch the chest fall. This is called an effective breath.

3 **If the chest does not rise**, reposition the child's head to make sure the airway is open; check the mouth for any obstructions. Try again up to five times. Stop as soon as you manage two effective breaths.

WARNING

- If you still cannot get the breaths in after five attempts, then go on to check for signs of circulation.
- If you cannot get the breaths in and you know the child choked on something don't check circulation, begin CPR straightaway (opposite).

4 **Check for signs of circulation**. Put your ear close to the child's face again and look down the chest for signs of movement, breathing, or coughing. Look for no more than 10 seconds.

5 **If you see signs of circulation**, continue with rescue breaths for ONE minute – at a rate of about 20 breaths per minute – then repeat the circulation check. If the child starts breathing, place her in the recovery position (p.19) while waiting for the ambulance.

6 **If there are no signs** of circulation, start giving CPR (cardiopulmonary resuscitation, see opposite), in order to maintain some blood circulation for the child.

giving a toddler CPR

CPR (cardiopulmonary resuscitation) involves giving chest compressions and rescue breaths. It is necessary if the toddler shows no signs of blood circulation. Through CPR it is possible to maintain some blood circulation.

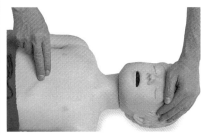

1 Place the child on a firm surface. Find the child's lowest rib and run your fingertips along the line of the ribs until you reach the central breastbone.

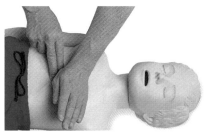

2 Put your middle finger on the breastbone and the forefinger beside it. Place the heel of your other hand against your fingertips.

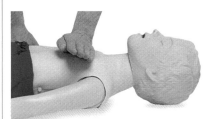

3 Make sure your shoulder is directly over your hand and, keeping your arm straight and fingertips off the chest, press down sharply on the chest to depress it by about one third of its depth. Release the pressure (but don't remove your hand). Repeat this five times at a rate of about 100 compressions a minute.

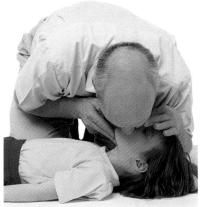

4 Then give the child one rescue breath as described opposite.

CONTINUE CHEST COMPRESSIONS AND RESCUE BREATHS

Continue giving five chest compressions and one rescue breath at this rate until the ambulance arrives, the child starts moving or breathing, or you're too exhausted to keep going.

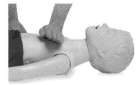

five compressions

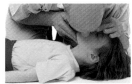

one rescue breath

BREATHING DIFFICULTIES

Any restrictions to a baby or child's ability to breathe must be treated at once to maintain the supply of oxygen to the body.

choking baby

Choking can happen when a foreign body becomes lodged in the throat and blocks the airway or causes muscular spasm. A baby can choke on a piece of food that is too big, or on something she's put in her mouth. You must act quickly or breathing could stop. Use this method on babies under 12 months.

SYMPTOMS

- Difficulty breathing, often makes high-pitched wheezing sound
- Trying to cry but makes very strange noises, or none at all
- Baby starts to turn blue, especially obvious around the lips

WARNING

- Never put your fingers in a baby's mouth to feel for an object you can't see.
- If the baby becomes unconscious, stop and go to p.16. Then follow the treatment for an unconscious baby.

1 If the baby becomes distressed, lay her face down along your forearm, supporting her head and neck (place her over your lap if she is too heavy).

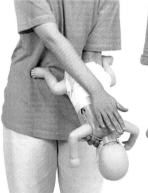 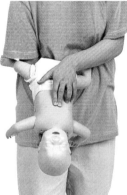 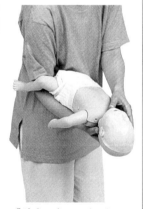

2 Give up to five sharp slaps on the back with the flat of your hand. Turn her over on to your other arm and check her mouth. Pick out anything you can see clearly.

3 If the obstruction is still there, put two fingers on the lower part of the breastbone about a finger's breadth below the nipple line and give up to five thrusts pressing downwards and forwards – towards the mouth (chest thrusts). Then check the mouth again.

4 If the obstruction is still there, repeat five backslaps followed by five chest thrusts. Do this up to three times (checking mouth between each set). then call an ambulance if someone hasn't already done this for you. Continue until help arrives.

choking toddler

Young children can easily choke on a piece of food that they haven't chewed properly, or because they have a habit of putting little things such as toys into their mouths. Use the following technique on toddlers over 12 months.

1 **Encourage the child to cough** if she can, as this is the most effective way to relieve the blockage.

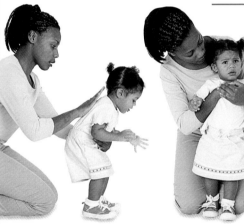

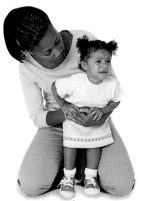

2 **If the child starts to become weak**, stand or kneel beside her and help her to bend forwards. Support her around the waist with one hand and give her up to five sharp slaps on the upper part of her back with your other hand. Check her mouth and pick out anything that you can see clearly.

3 **Give chest thrusts** if the child is still choking. Stand or kneel behind the child. Make a fist with one hand and hold your fist thumb inwards against the lower half of the child's breastbone. Grasp your fist with your other hand and pull it sharply inwards and upwards. Do this up to five times. Look inside her mouth again.

4 **Try abdominal thrusts** if the child is still choking. This time place your fist thumb inwards against the child's upper abdomen and pull sharply inwards and upwards up to five times. Look in her mouth again.

5 **If the blockage** remains, repeat the sequence of back slaps, chest thrusts, and abdominal thrusts up to three times, then call an ambulance. Continue the sequence until help arrives.

asthma

A common chronic illness in childhood, asthma can be an allergic reaction and is brought on by various triggers. The symptoms of asthma – cough, wheezing, and shortness of breath – are caused by narrowing of the air passages (bronchi). An asthma attack can be very frightening for a child, because the feeling of suffocation can cause panic, making breathing even more difficult.

SYMPTOMS
- Difficulty in breathing
- Wheezing when breathing out
- Coughing
- Tiredness and anxiety
- Blue tinge on face and lips

WARNING
- Call an ambulance immediately if it's your child's first attack, or if the attack is severe and doesn't respond to treatment.

1 **Stay as calm** as you can so you can calm your child – he may be frightened by what's happening.

2 **Give your child** a puff on a reliever or inhaler if he has one.

3 **If the attack happens** when your child is in bed, sit him up, propped up with pillows. Otherwise, have him sitting up straight on a chair and leaning forwards against a table or the back of another chair to take the weight off his chest. This allows his chest muscles to force air out more efficiently.

GIVING ASTHMA MEDICATION TO BABIES AND YOUNG CHILDREN

1 **Fit the inhaler** and spacer together as instructed by your doctor. Check that they're working by shaking and depressing the inhaler.

2 **Hold your child** on your lap. Put the mouthpiece in your child's mouth or the mask over your baby's face.

3 **Squeeze the inhaler** and hold the spacer in place until your child has taken five deep breaths. This should ensure that he's inhaled all the drug.

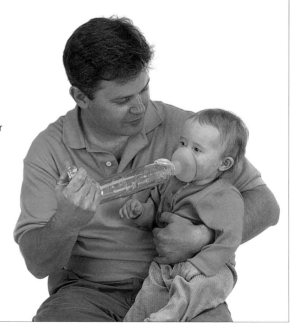

croup

Croup is the name given to the sound made when air is breathed in through a constricted windpipe, past inflamed vocal cords. It usually happens only in young children, who are susceptible because their air passages (bronchi) are narrow and become blocked with mucus when inflamed – often because of a virus such as a common cold, or an infection such as bronchitis. Croup can also be caused by an inhaled foreign object. If croup is severe and accompanied by fever, call an ambulance because in rare cases it could be epiglottitis.

The first attack of croup can come on quickly, usually at night, and it may last a couple of hours. Your child will have a croaking cough and laboured breathing.

SYMPTOMS

- Croaking cough
- Difficulty and wheezing when breathing in
- Face colour becomes greyish or blue

WARNING

- Check with your doctor immediately if your child's skin turns grey or blue and he has to fight for breath. Speak to your doctor as soon as possible to tell him that your child has had an attack of croup.

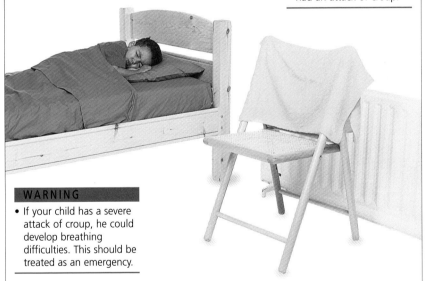

WARNING

- If your child has a severe attack of croup, he could develop breathing difficulties. This should be treated as an emergency.

1 **Stay calm** and try to calm your child so that he won't panic and make his breathing more difficult.

2 **Moist air** will soothe your child's air passages. If the air outside is cool and damp, take him to the window and get him to take a deep breath of air, or take him into the bathroom and turn on the hot taps to build up a steamy atmosphere.

3 **Prop your child up** in bed with pillows or hold him on your lap. It will be easier for him to breathe if he is sitting up. A damp towel near a radiator will help keep the air in the room moist.

suffocation and strangulation

Both of these emergencies can prevent a child breathing. In strangulation something caught around the child's neck constricts the air passages. In suffocation, an obstruction prevents air entering the body. This could be something over the face or a weight on the chest or abdomen. Smoke and fumes can also prevent air getting to the body.

1 Remove whatever is stopping the child breathing. If a child is suffocating, simply removing the obstruction may allow her to breathe again. If a child is hanging, make sure you support her body while releasing her neck.

2 Open the airway. Put your hand on the child's forehead and tilt the head back. Lift the chin with two fingers of your other hand to open the airway.

3 Look and listen for breathing for 10 seconds.

4 If she's not breathing, give rescue breaths (p.17; p.20).

5 If she is breathing, place her in the recovery position (pp.18–19) and call an ambulance. Stay with her and continue to check her breathing and pulse until help arrives.

Hold in the recovery position

PREVENTION

• Don't put a pillow in the cot for a baby under 12 months: it could suffocate her. If you want to raise her head, put a pillow under the mattress.

• Don't use a duvet for a baby under 12 months old. She could get trapped under the duvet and suffocate.

• Cot toys should not have strings that are longer than 30cm (12in).

• Keep plastic bags out of reach. If a toy comes wrapped in a plastic bag, unwrap it for your child and throw away the bag.

• Don't use cot bumpers and never leave plastic covers on mattresses.

drowning

A baby or toddler can drown in just 2.5cm (1in) of water, for instance if she falls in her bath or slips into a paddling pool. Even a bucket of water can be a danger. If a drowning child isn't rescued quickly she'll be asphyxiated.

IF THE CHILD IS UNCONSCIOUS

1 **Get the child** out of the water as quickly as possible. Hold her with her head lower than her chest to reduce the risk of inhaling water or vomit.

2 **Lay her down** on her back on a coat, blanket, or rug. Check her condition (p.16 for baby; p.19 for toddler). Be prepared to begin resuscitation if necessary. You may have to breathe more firmly and slowly than normal in order to get the chest to rise – water in the lungs can increase the resistance to rescue breathing.

3 **As soon as** the child is breathing, remove her wet clothes and cover her with a dry towel or blanket. Place her in the recovery position (pp.18–19) and call an ambulance.

4 **Even if the child** appears to have recovered fully, call an ambulance. Any water that has entered the lungs can cause irritation and the air passages may begin to swell some hours later. The child may also need to be treated for hypothermia.

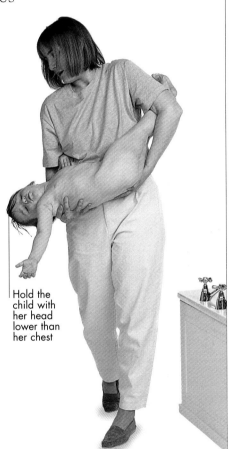

Hold the child with her head lower than her chest

PREVENTION

• Never leave a baby or toddler alone in a bath: she could go under the water and drown, even in 2.5cm (1in) of water. If you leave the room, take your baby with you.

• If you have a pond or swimming pool and your child is under two years, drain the water, cover it, or fence it off.

• Never leave a baby or toddler to play alone in or near water.

• If you have a paddling pool in your garden, empty it out after use.

• Fit any water-collecting devices, such as butts, with a close-fitting lid so that children cannot fall inside.

chest wound

A wound to the chest can cause serious damage, particularly to the lungs. A child may have breathing problems, a collapsed lung, and shock after a chest injury. Most important is to make an airtight seal around the wound to stop air entering the cavity while you wait for help.

WARNING
If your child becomes unconscious
• Assess his condition.
• Be prepared to resuscitate.
• Check for shock.

1 **Call an ambulance**.

2 **Holding the palm** of your hand over the wound, prop your child up in a semi-upright position.

3 **Place a clean pad** or a sterile dressing over the wound and tape it securely on three sides.

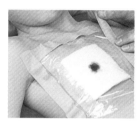

4 **To seal the wound**, cover the dressing with kitchen film, held in place with tape on three sides.

5 **Keep checking** your child's condition (see monitoring vital signs p.12) and be prepared to resuscitate. Check for signs of shock (p.30).

6 **If your child becomes unconscious** and you need to put him in the recovery position (pp.18–19), lie him on his injured side.

winding

"Winding" is a temporary breathing problem caused by a blow to the upper abdomen which stuns a local nerve junction.

Sit your child down, loosen any clothing around his waist or chest and comfort him. He should soon recover.

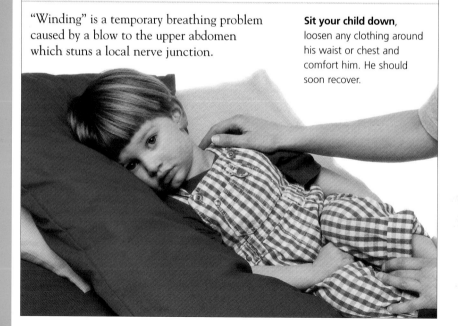

extreme allergic reaction

Also known as anaphylactic shock, this is a severe and life-threatening allergic reaction that may develop within a few minutes of the injection of a particular drug, the sting of an insect or a sea creature, or eating a particular food. Nuts, for example, are known to cause anaphylactic shock. All the symptoms may come at once and the child may lose consciousness fast. This is a medical emergency so get help immediately.

SYMPTOMS

- High-pitched wheezing sound
- Attempts to cough
- Difficulty speaking then breathing
- Child begins to turn blue, especially visible around the lips

1 **Call an ambulance**. If your child has had this reaction before, she'll have medication to take in case of more attacks. Use this as soon as the attack starts, following your doctor's instructions carefully.

2 **Help your child** into a comfortable position that most relieves her breathing difficulty and loosen any tight clothing at her neck and waist. Soothe and reassure her while you wait for medical help to arrive.

3 **If your child** loses consciousness, open her airways, check her breathing and be prepared to begin rescue breathing (p.17 baby; p.20 toddler).

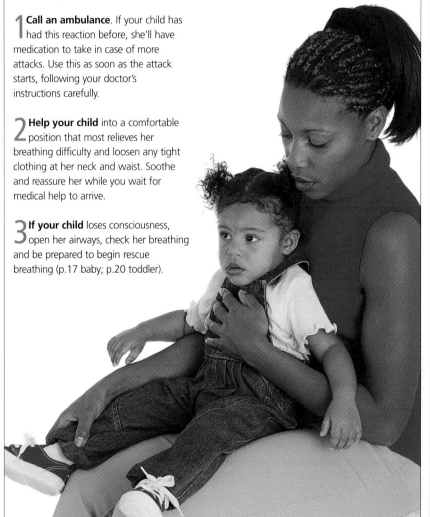

SHOCK

In a medical context shock refers to a dangerous condition in which the blood circulatory system fails because there's not enough fluid in the body. The most common causes are severe bleeding and burns.

treating shock

After an initial adrenaline rush, the body withdraws blood from the skin to serve the vital organs – the oxygen supply to the brain drops.

1 **If possible, ask someone else to call an ambulance** while you stay with your child. Lay your child down, keeping his head low to improve the blood supply to the brain. Treat any obvious cause such as serious bleeding.

2 **Raise your child's legs** and support them with pillows or on a cushion on a pile of books.

3 **Loosen any tight clothing** at the neck, chest, and waist to make breathing easier.

4 **Cover your child with a blanket** or coat to keep him warm. Don't use a hot-water bottle or any other direct source of heat.

5 **Keep talking to your child** and checking his condition as you wait for the ambulance. If your child loses consciousness, open his airway, check his breathing, and be prepared to begin rescue breathing (p.17 baby; p.20 toddler).

6 **Don't give your child anything** to eat or drink. If he does complain of thirst, just moisten his lips with water.

SYMPTOMS

Early signs of shock
- Pale, cold, sweaty skin that is often greyish looking, especially around the lips.
- Rapid pulse, becoming weaker
- Shallow, fast breathing

Symptoms as shock progresses:
- Fontanelle is drawn in
- Restlessness, yawning, sighing
- Thirst
- Loss of consciousness

SHOCK IN BABIES

If your baby is suffering from shock, hold him on your lap while you loosen his clothing and comfort him. Otherwise treat as for toddlers (above). Check your baby's head – an important symptom of shock in babies under two years is a drawn-in fontanelle, the soft spot on top of the skull where the bones are still not joined.

INTERNAL BLEEDING

Shock can be caused by internal bleeding after an injury. If your child develops any of the symptoms listed above, even though he shows no obvious signs of injury, if he complains of severe pain in the chest, or is unusually quiet after an accident, treat him as described above and get him to a hospital as soon as possible.

WOUNDS AND BLEEDING

Cuts and grazes are rarely serious and, unless infected, can be dealt with at home. Severe external or internal bleeding, however, can lead to shock and loss of consciousness, and should be treated as emergencies.

cuts and grazes

Superficial cuts should only need cleaning and dressing. A jagged deeper cut may require stitches. If a cut is deep or dirty, there's also a risk of tetanus.

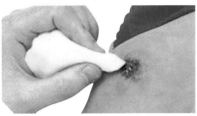

1 Sit your child down on a chair or hold your baby in your lap. Using a gauze pad or a very soft brush, gently wash the graze with soap and water. Wipe away from the wound and use a clean piece of gauze for each wipe.

2 If there are any particles of dirt or gravel embedded in the wound, try to remove them. This may cause more bleeding so press on the wound with a clean pad to stop bleeding.

3 Using a plaster large enough to cover the wound and surrounding area, dress the cut or graze. Don't put cotton wool or any other fluffy material on the wound. It'll stick and delay healing.

4 If you can't remove all the dirt from a wound, take your child to hospital.

bruises

Unsteady on their feet, toddlers often get bruises from knocks and falls. These are rarely serious but resting, cooling, and holding up the affected part will soothe any pain.

1 To reduce swelling and pain, hold one of the suggested cold compresses (right) against the area for 30 minutes. If necessary, hold the compress in place with a bandage.

2 Using a clean gauze pad or a very soft brush, gently wash the graze with soap and running water if you can.

A bag of frozen peas, wrapped in a light towel.

Plastic bag of ice – fill two-thirds full with ice cubes. Add a little salt to help the ice melt, then seal. Wrap in a towel.

A soft cloth, wrung out in cold water and replaced every 10 minutes.

mouth wound

Don't rinse the mouth out or you may disturb a blood clot. Call a doctor if the bleeding hasn't stopped in 20 minutes.

1 **Sit your child with her head** over a bowl and tell her to let the blood dribble out of her mouth.

2 **Place** a clean pad over the wound. Press it between your thumb and forefinger for 10 minutes. Repeat if necessary.

knocked-out tooth

If a child's tooth gets knocked out, try to find it so that you know it hasn't been swallowed or inhaled. Milk teeth cannot be replanted, but you'll still need immediate dental advice and a check-up for your child.

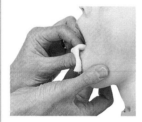

1 **Sit your child down** and place a clean pad over the gum. The pad should be higher than the teeth to make it easier to hold in place.

2 **Ask your child** to bite hard on the pad. You may need to hold the pad in place for a very young child.

3 **Take your child** to the dentist and ask the dentist to check the gum.

nosebleed

A nosebleed happens if the small area of blood vessels just inside the nose ruptures. It can be caused by nose-blowing, sneezing, a blow to the nose, picking the nose or a foreign object in the nose. Nosebleeds aren't serious, but if your child has frequent nosebleeds which are hard to stop, check with your doctor.

WARNING
- If a nosebleed lasts more than 30 minutes or if your child has had a blow to the head and there's watery discharge from her nose, call an ambulance.

1 **Sit your child with her** head forward over a basin. Tell her to breathe through her mouth. Applying firm pressure to both nostrils, grip the fleshy part of her nose and squeeze for 10 minutes.

2 **Let your child spit out** any blood in her mouth. If the bleeding hasn't stopped, pinch again for 10 minutes. Repeat if necessary.

3 **If the bleeding stops, gently** clean your child's nose with cotton wool and warm water. Let her rest. Don't let her blow or pick her nose for at least three hours or it might bleed again.

eye wound

Any injury to the eye should be treated as soon as possible since it could have long-term consequences for your child's sight. For treating foreign objects in the eye, see p.45. For a chemical burn to the eye, see p.37.

1 **Hold your baby** or lie your child down with her head on your lap. Encourage her to keep her eyes still.

2 **Cover the injured eye** with a sterile dressing.

3 **Call an ambulance.** Keep your child lying on her back until help arrives.

ear wound

A cut to the outside of the ear can bleed profusely and be very painful. Never try to insert anything into your child's ear to clean a wound.

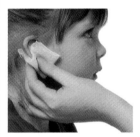
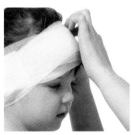

1 **Using a piece** of clean gauze, gently pinch the wound to stop the bleeding. Hold for 10 minutes.

2 **Cover the ear** with a sterile dressing and bandage it in place.

3 **Stitches** may be needed for a wound made by an earring being torn out, so take your child to hospital.

blisters

A blister is a fluid-filled bubble of skin that is caused by burns, friction, or exposure to extremes of heat and cold. Protect blisters but never burst them yourself as this can cause infection.

1 **Clean the blister** carefully with soap and water. Rinse and dry the area well.

2 **Protect the area with a plaster** that has a pad large enough to cover the whole blister.

3 **If the blister does burst**, keep it clean and dry and cover it with a clean gauze dressing.

serious bleeding

Bleeding happens when any of the vessels that carry blood around the body is cut or torn. It can appear externally if the skin is damaged, but can also happen internally. Heavy bleeding is both serious and distressing and should be dealt with as an emergency. If too much blood is lost from the child's circulatory system, there won't be enough left to supply the body cells with oxygen, and shock and loss of consciousness can result. Treat bleeding quickly, as described below, and reassure your child.

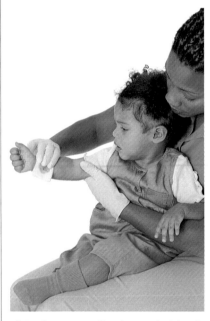

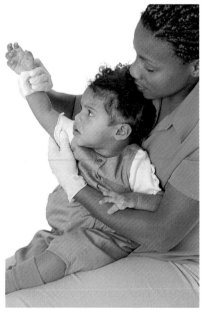

1 Apply pressure directly over the injured area. Use your fingers or the palm of your hand, or place a clean pad over the wound, and press against it. Press firmly enough to stop the wound bleeding.

2 Raise the injured part above the level of your child's heart. Cover the wound with a clean, non-fluffy dressing that is larger than the injury itself, still keeping the injury raised above the level of the heart. Don't use cotton wool or fluffy material that may stick to the injury.

3 Secure the dressing with a bandage, tied firmly over the injury, but not so tight as to cut off the blood supply. If any blood comes through the bandage, secure another dressing with a second bandage firmly on top. If bleeding comes through the second dressing, remove both and start again.

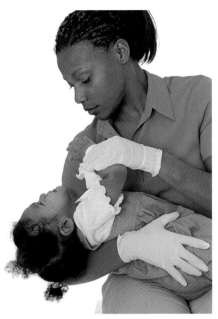

4 **Lay your child down**, still keeping the injury raised, and watch for any signs of shock (p.30).

5 **Get your child to a hospital** as soon as possible because she may need stitches. Either call an ambulance or get another adult to drive you while you sit with your child, continuing first aid if needed. Either hold your child in your arms, while keeping pressure on the injury, or lie your child down with her head low. Press on the wound for up to 10 minutes.

CARE OF AN AMPUTATED PART

It may be possible to reattach an amputated part such as a finger by microsurgery. It's vital to get the child and the amputated part to hospital as soon as possible.

1 **Apply direct pressure** to the injured area with a clean pad. If possible, raise the injury above the level of the heart.

2 **Cover the injury** with a bandage and tape it securely in place. Or use a finger bandage.

3 **Lay the child down** and call an ambulance. Tell the control officer what has happened.

4 **Put the amputated** part in a small plastic bag or wrap it in some kitchen film.

5 **Wrap the bag** in a soft cotton handkerchief or some gauze.

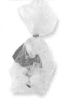

6 **Put the wrapped bag** in another plastic bag filled with ice cubes.

7 **Place the package** in another bag or a plastic container. Make sure it's clearly marked with your child's name and the date and time of injury before you hand it to ambulance or hospital personnel.

TREATING BURNS

Superficial burns are caused by contact with hot liquid or touching a hot surface and are the least serious type of burn. Deeper burns are more serious and cause fluid-filled blisters. Very deep burns are the most serious, as all layers of the skin are affected, but may be the least painful because the nerves are often damaged. If a fire has caused the burn, the smoke and hot air may also have affected your child's lungs and air passages. **A baby or young child with a burn should always be checked at hospital.**

burns

The larger the area of any burn, the greater the risk of severe shock (p.30) because of loss of body fluids. Remember that with soft, delicate skin, even hot bathwater can burn a baby, so always check its temperature before bathing your child.

WARNING

Burns to the mouth and throat
- These can be particularly dangerous as they can cause swelling of the air passages and suffocation. Loosen any clothing around the neck and call an ambulance immediately.

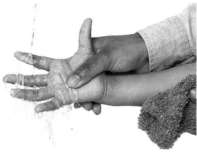

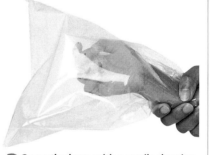

1 Cool the affected area immediately. Hold it under cool running water for at least 10 minutes. If there's no water available, you can use a non-flammable liquid such as milk.

2 While cooling, remove any constricting clothing from the affected area before it begins to swell. Cut round any material that's sticking to the child's skin. If your child is still in pain, cool the burned area again. Be careful not to touch the burned area or burst any blisters. Don't overcool your child or you could cause hypothermia (p.50).

3 Cover the burn with a sterile dressing or clean, non-fluffy material to protect it from infection. Use a pillowcase or a sheet for a large area or put a clean plastic bag or kitchen film over a burned hand or foot.

4 Check your child for any sign of shock and don't give him anything to eat or drink. Keep him warm to guard against hypothermia.

5 If your child loses consciousness, open his airways, check his breathing and be prepared to begin rescue breathing (p.17 baby; p.20 toddler).

if your child's clothing is on fire

If your child's clothing should catch fire, the first priority is to stop him moving. Any rapid movement will make the flames worse.

1 Stop him running around in a panic because this will fan the flames. Lie him on the floor with the burning side uppermost.

2 Wrap him in a heavy woollen coat or blanket to stifle the flames. Never use nylon – it's inflammable.

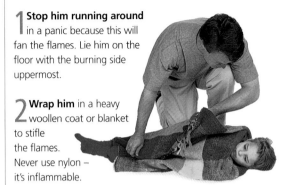

WARNING
• Don't remove any clothing. It may be sticking to the skin and moving it will cause further damage.

3 Roll him on the ground to put out the flames. Douse him with water if you have some, or another non-flammable liquid.

chemical burn on the skin

Household items such as oven cleaner or paint stripper can cause burns that are serious but develop more slowly than burns caused by heat. Signs include stinging pain, redness or staining followed by blistering and peeling.

1 Follow the procedure for burns but cool under running water for 20 minutes and protect yourself by wearing rubber gloves.

2 Make sure you know what caused your child's burn so that you can tell the doctors when you reach hospital.

chemical burn to eye

Accidental splashes of chemicals in the eye can cause damage or even blindness. The child will have severe pain in his eye, which will appear red and will be watering. Your child will also find it difficult to open his eye. You mustn't let your child rub or touch his eye, to avoid the chemical being spread to other parts of his face.

1 Wash out the chemical immediately. Hold your child's head over a basin, the unaffected eye uppermost, and run cold water over the affected eye for 20 minutes. Wear rubber gloves to protect yourself. If it is difficult to hold your child over a basin, pour water from a jug over the eye.

2 When the eye is well rinsed, cover it with a clean pad until you get to hospital.

electrical burn

An electric shock can cause burns not only at the point where the current enters the body, but also where it leaves. The burns may look small but they are often deep so carry a serious risk of infection.

Make sure that the contact is broken before you touch your child or you'll get a shock yourself. If you can't switch off the power, find something that won't conduct electricity, such as a broom or a plastic tube, and push your child away from the source of the power. Make sure that your hands and whatever you're using are dry and that you're not standing on anything that's wet or made of metal.

1 **If your child has lost consciousness**, open her airway, check her breathing, and be prepared to begin rescue breaths (p.17 baby; p.20 toddler).

Break the electrical contact before touching the child

2 **Cool the burn** by holding the affected area under cold running water for at least 10 minutes.

3 **Cover the burn** with clean, non-fluffy material or with a clean plastic bag which you can tape in place.

HOW TO PREVENT ELECTRICAL ACCIDENTS

• Wire plugs safely and check you have the right fuse.

• Check flexes aren't worn and make sure there are no protruding wires.

• Put dummy covers in unused sockets.

• Don't leave trailing wires where a child can reach or fall over them.

• Fit a circuit-breaking device.

sunburn

Children's skin is very sensitive to the damaging ultraviolet rays of sunlight, and overexposure to the sun in infancy greatly increases the long-term risk of skin cancer. Sunburn over large areas of the skin can be serious.

TREATING SUNBURN

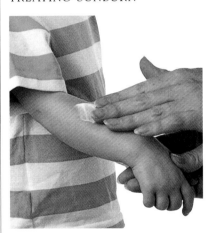

1 **Get your child into the shade** or a cool room. Give her a cool drink.

2 **Soothe any red skin** with calamine lotion or after-sun cream.

3 **Keep your child out of direct sun** for at least 48 hours.

4 **If she has any blistering** or shows signs of heatstroke (p.51), call a doctor.

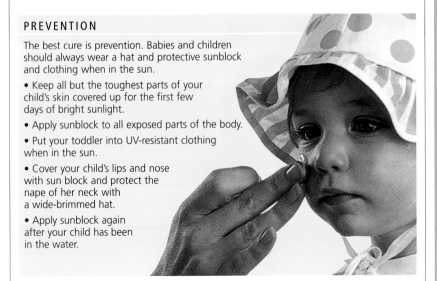

PREVENTION

The best cure is prevention. Babies and children should always wear a hat and protective sunblock and clothing when in the sun.

- Keep all but the toughest parts of your child's skin covered up for the first few days of bright sunlight.

- Apply sunblock to all exposed parts of the body.

- Put your toddler into UV-resistant clothing when in the sun.

- Cover your child's lips and nose with sun block and protect the nape of her neck with a wide-brimmed hat.

- Apply sunblock again after your child has been in the water.

HEAD INJURY

A head injury causing unconsciousness, dizziness, or vomiting is always serious. Bleeding or clear discharge from the nose or ear after a head injury is a sign of skull fracture and is an emergency. If the child has fallen from a height and hit his head, spine injury is also possible (p.49).

WARNING
- All children with head injuries should be seen by a doctor.
- Never shake a baby. It can cause head injury.

scalp wounds

This type of injury often looks more alarming than it is. Scalp wounds tend to bleed profusely and bruises can be large because there are so many blood vessels running close to the surface in the scalp. The sight of so much blood can be very frightening for both you and your child.

WARNING
- A soft area on the skull and blood showing in the white of the eye may indicate skull fracture – see compression, opposite.

IF YOUR CHILD IS CONSCIOUS

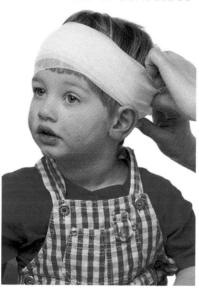

1 **Press a wound dressing** or clean pad against the wound for about 10 minutes.

2 **Secure the dressing with a bandage** to help keep an even pressure. If blood comes through the dressing pad, cover the pad with another one. If it comes through the second dressing, remove both and start again as there won't be enough pressure.

3 **Lie your child down**, keeping his head and shoulders slightly raised.

4 **Get your child to hospital**. Monitor your child's vital signs, level of consciousness, pulse, and breathing (p.12). Watch especially for any signs of his condition deteriorating – this could indicate possible compression injury, see opposite.

IF YOUR CHILD LOSES CONSCIOUSNESS

Open his airway, check his breathing, and be prepared to begin rescue breathing (p.17 baby; p.20 toddler).

If you suspect that he has injured his back, open his airway using the jaw thrust (see spinal injury, p.49). Don't tilt his head.

concussion

This is caused by a blow to the head that "shakes" the brain within the skull, and it is characterized by a short period of unconsciousness or dazed feeling after the injury. The symptoms may not appear right away but they are always followed by recovery. If the child deteriorates again it is not concussion.

SYMPTOMS

• Head injury
• Short period of unconsciousness, then complete recovery of consciousness
• Child may feel dizzy or sick on recovery
• Possible loss of memory of anything that happened just before the event
• Mild headache

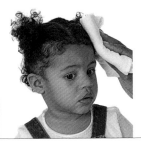

1 **Place a cold compress** against the injury or treat bleeding for a scalp wound.

2 **Sit or lie your child down**. Check her level of consciousness (p.12) and make a note of it.

3 **Go to hospital** or call an ambulance.

4 **If your child's** condition deteriorates, treat as for unconsciousness (p.16 baby; p.19 toddler) or monitor her vital signs until help arrives.

compression

Potentially very serious, this is caused by bleeding under the skull that presses on the brain, by skull fracture, especially if the bone presses against the brain, or by swelling of the brain tissues after a head injury. Urgent medical attention, and almost certainly an operation, is needed to prevent permanent brain damage. Compression may not develop until some hours after a head injury, so monitor your child carefully.

1 **Sit her down with her head and shoulders raised**. Treat any wounds. Check her level of consciousness (p.12) and make a note of it.

2 **If she becomes unconscious**, treat as described on pp.16–18 for babies or pp.19–21 for toddlers. Call an ambulance. Be prepared to begin rescue breathing if necessary. If she's breathing, monitor her level of consciousness, breathing, and pulse until help arrives.

SYMPTOMS

• Head injury
• Clear discharge from the nose or ears, indicating possible skull fracture
• Severe headache
• Deteriorating level of consciousness, eventually leading to complete unconsciousness
• Pupils of eyes may be different sizes
• High temperature and flushed face
• Breathing may be noisy then becomes very slow
• Weakness or even loss of movement down one side of the body

BITES AND STINGS

Most animal bites are caused by a child's boisterous teasing of a household pet, though in rare instances, pets have been known to make unprovoked attacks on infants. As a precaution, watch your baby or toddler when there are cats, dogs or other pets around. Don't leave a baby sleeping outside in an open pram unprotected from insects. Many prams do have mosquito nets fitted. Always keep a close eye on your child in the garden or on the beach.

animal bites

Being bitten by an animal can be traumatic for your child, but bites from domestic pets such as dogs and cats aren't usually serious. If the bite or scratch is deep, bacteria from the animal's teeth or claws will be lodged in the wound, making infection likely. Most animal bites can be treated at home with comfort and simple first aid, but more serious bite wounds will require hospital treatment.

WARNING

- If your child is bitten by an animal in a country where there is rabies or if it's possible that the animal has been smuggled into the UK, take your child to hospital for anti-rabies treatment.

IF THE BITE IS SUPERFICIAL

1 **Calm your child** and reassure him if he's frightened.

2 **Wash the wound** with warm water and soap. Rinse under running water for at least five minutes to remove any blood, saliva, or dirt.

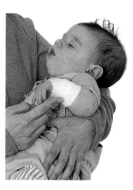

3 **Dry the wound** gently but carefully with a clean pad or tissue. Apply a plaster or sterile dressing.

4 **Check with your doctor** as soon as possible to make sure that the bite isn't infected or deep enough to carry the risk of tetanus. Make sure your child is protected against tetanus.

IF THE BITE IS SERIOUS AND DEEP

1 **Cover the wound** with a clean dressing or pad and apply pressure with your hand to stop the bleeding. If possible, lift the affected part above your child's heart.

2 **Place a clean dressing** over the wound and bandage it in place.

3 **Take your child** to hospital or call an ambulance. He will need treatment as soon as possible to prevent infection.

insect stings

Bee and wasp stings are painful but rarely serious, unless your child has an extreme allergic reaction (p.29). A sting appears as a raised white area on an inflamed area of skin.

1 **Calm your child** and encourage him to keep as still as possible to slow down the rate of spreading of the poison.

2 **If the sting is still in the skin**, brush it off or scrape it off with a credit card or fingernail. Don't squeeze the sac at the top of the skin or try to remove the sting with tweezers or you'll force more poison into your child.

3 **To reduce the pain and swelling**, apply a cold compress (p.31) to the area. Keep it in place for about 10 minutes until the pain lessens.

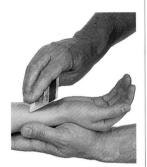

STING IN THE MOUTH

A sting in the mouth can cause swelling and lead to breathing problems, so get medical help quickly.

1 **Reduce any swelling** by giving your child cold water to drink or an ice cube to suck, unless he's under 12 months. Call the doctor.

2 **If the area swells** quickly and your child is finding it difficult to breathe, call an ambulance.

sting from a sea creature

Jellyfish, sea anemones, and other sea creatures have stinging cells that release venom when touched. Most cause only an itchy rash, but some are highly venomous and their sting can be much more serious, even fatal.

1 **Apply a cold compress** to the affected area and hold it in place for 10 minutes. If possible, raise the affected part.

2 **If the sting** is very red and painful, take your child to hospital.

3 **If spines** from a sea creature are embedded in your child's foot, soak the foot in hot water for 30 minutes or more to loosen them. If the spines don't come out or the foot swells, take your child to hospital.

4 **If a jellyfish stings** your child, pour salt water or vinegar over the injury to neutralize the stinging cells. Bandage the limb above the wound and call an ambulance.

FOREIGN OBJECTS

Growing children are naturally curious and they love to put things in their mouths, ears, and even up their noses. They're still learning what's safe to touch so injuries involving foreign objects are quite common.

splinter

A splinter is a tiny sliver of material that becomes embedded in or under the skin. It may be wood, metal, glass, a thorn, or a prickle. Deep splinters can carry the risk of tetanus infection so check your child is protected.

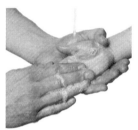

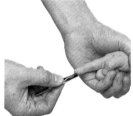

1 **Wash the skin** around the splinter with soap and warm water.

2 **Take a pair of tweezers** and sterilize them by passing the ends through a blue flame. Allow them to cool, but don't touch or wipe the ends.

3 **Grip the splinter** with the tweezers as close to the skin as possible. Pull it out at the same angle it went in.

4 **Squeeze the wound** to make it bleed and flush out any dirt. Clean the area again. Dry it well and cover with a plaster.

WARNING

- If the splinter breaks or you cannot get it out, take your child to the doctor.
- Take your child to the doctor if the splinter is glass.
- Do not poke at the splinter with a needle.
- If the splinter is dirty or contaminated with garden material, check with your doctor about a tetanus inoculation for your child.

foreign object in ear

Children often push objects such as beads into their ears. Anything stuck in the ear must be removed or it can cause infection or damage the eardrum.

1 **If your child gets** a hard object stuck in his ear, don't try to remove it, even if you can see what it is. Take your child to hospital where it can be removed safely.

2 **If an insect flies** into your child's ear, sit him down or hold him with the affected ear uppermost. Gently pour warm water into the ear. The insect should float out.

3 **If you can't remove** an insect, take your child to hospital. Reassure your child that the insect will come out.

foreign object in eye

If you can see something moving over the white part of the eye you can try to remove it. If it's embedded in the eyeball or is on the coloured part of the eye (the iris), don't touch it – take your child to hospital.

1 **Look to see** if the foreign object is moving or embedded in the eye. Sit your child facing the light. Ask him to look up, down, left, and right and look at all of the eye.

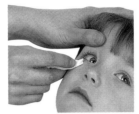

2 **If you spot** the object, try to flush it out. Put some clean water in a jug, tilt the head back, and pour water into the corner of the eye so the water washes over it.

3 **If this doesn't work**, use a damp cotton wool swab or handkerchief to lift the object off the eye.

4 **If the object** is under the eyelid, wrap your child in a towel to restrain him. Then carefully lift the upper eyelid down over the lower eyelid to clear anything caught under it.

5 **If you cannot remove** the object, cover your child's eye with a clean pad and take him to hospital.

foreign object in nose

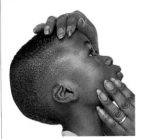

Something pushed into your child's nose may not be noticed at first, but after two or three days it will cause a nosebleed or smelly blood-stained discharge. Your child may have difficult or noisy breathing and swelling of the nose.

1 **Encourage your child** to breathe through his mouth and check his nose.

2 **Don't try** to remove the object yourself. Take your child to hospital.

swallowed foreign object

Babies and toddlers explore the world with their mouths so often swallow small objects.

1 **Try to find** out what your child has swallowed. A small smooth object such as a pebble or coin shouldn't cause any problems.

2 **If you don't know** what your child has swallowed or the object is large or sharp, take your child to hospital. Don't give him anything to eat or drink.

BONES, JOINTS AND MUSCLES

In babies and toddlers, it can be difficult to tell the difference between broken bones and muscle sprains or strains. Always treat such injury as a possible broken bone and get the child to hospital for X-rays.

broken bones

Children's bones are like young, bendy twigs on a tree; they don't snap as easily as the harder bones of an adult. A greenstick fracture is most common in children, in which the bone bends and splits but doesn't break, and there is little damage in the surrounding tissue. Other types include simple fractures (the bone breaks cleanly in one place) and compound fractures (the bone breaks in more than one place). Either can damage blood vessels and muscles around the break.

A broken bone needs prompt treatment by a doctor, as it must be positioned correctly and any external wounds covered to minimize the risk of infection.

1 **Reassure your child**, and encourage her to stay as still as possible. If she's moved unnecessarily, the ends of any broken bones can damage surrounding blood vessels and nerves.

2 **Support the joints** above and below the injury to prevent further movement. Initially support them by hand, while someone gets cushions or rolled blankets to place around the injury and minimize the risk of movement. Don't try to straighten the broken limb.

3 **Get your child to hospital** as soon as possible. If the injury is on an arm or hand you can take your child by car provided you have help – one person to hold the child while the other drives. If your child has an injury to her leg, or she can't bend her elbow, call an ambulance as she may need to be carried on a stretcher.

4 **If a bone end has broken** through the skin, or there is a wound leading to the break, cover it with a wound dressing or drape a piece of gauze over the top to prevent infection. Don't try to clean the wound and don't touch the injury.

WARNING

- Never try to straighten a broken limb. If possible, support it with cushions or a sling.
- Don't move your child unless you have to get her to a safer place.

SYMPTOMS

- Swelling around the site of the injury
- Bruising around the site of the injury
- Possible deformation of the affected area
- Inability to move the affected area normally or without pain
- Pain

5 **If your child's injury needs extra support** you can "splint" the affected part, by securing it to a neighbouring uninjured part. For example, bandage an injured finger to the next one, Support an arm injury with a sling (see opposite) and provide extra support for a leg injury by securing the injured leg to the other one at the joints. Triangular bandages folded lengthways make useful supports.

arm or hand injury

A fall onto an outstretched hand can injure collarbones and shoulders, while a direct blow to the arm can cause a break or a greenstick fracture. A good way to keep your child's limb or joint still until an ambulance arrives is with a sling.

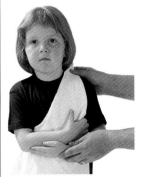 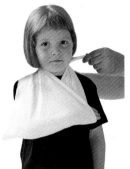 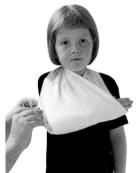

1 **Hold the child's injured** arm across her chest. Slide a triangular bandage between her arm and her chest so that the longest edge of the bandage is parallel to her uninjured side.

2 **Bring the lower half** of the bandage up over the injured arm and take the point around the back of your child's neck. Tie the end together in a knot over the hollow above her collarbone.

3 **Tuck the two ends** of the bandage under the knot – it's more comfortable. Fold the bandage over at the child's elbow and fix it in place with a safety pin. Get your child to hospital.

leg injury

Keep your child as still as possible while an ambulance is called. Don't take her to hospital yourself – she will need a stretcher. Your child could go into shock (p.30), especially if the thigh bone is broken.

Support the joints
Sit or lie your child down, and encourage her to stay still. Hold the joints above and below the injured area to prevent any movement. Support her leg with cushions or blankets and call an ambulance.

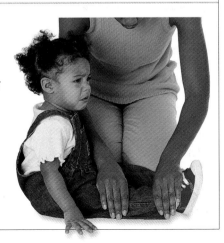

sprains and strains

A sprain is the tearing of the tough, strap-like structures called ligaments that support a joint. It's caused by a sudden overstretching or twisting action, and swelling, pain, and bruising can result. If no ligaments are torn and only muscle fibres are overstretched, this is a strain. It's often hard to tell what an injury is without an X-ray, so if in doubt, treat as a break (p.46). Strains and sprains should be first treated by the **"RICE"** procedure below.

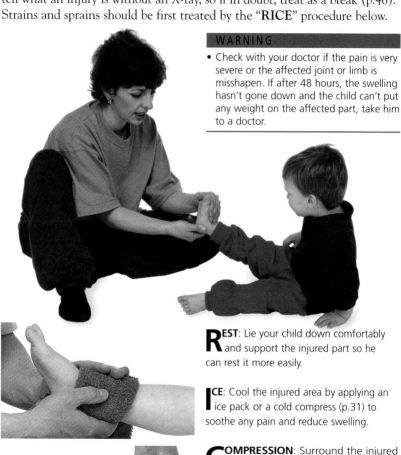

WARNING

• Check with your doctor if the pain is very severe or the affected joint or limb is misshapen. If after 48 hours, the swelling hasn't gone down and the child can't put any weight on the affected part, take him to a doctor.

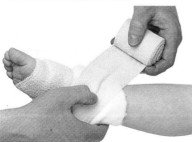

REST: Lie your child down comfortably and support the injured part so he can rest it more easily.

ICE: Cool the injured area by applying an ice pack or a cold compress (p.31) to soothe any pain and reduce swelling.

COMPRESSION: Surround the injured part with soft padding such as cotton wool and secure it with a bandage tight enough to apply gentle pressure (compression). Check the circulation beyond the bandaging.

ELEVATION: Raise the injured part to reduce the flow of blood to the area. This will help reduce bruising.

spine injury

If you suspect that your child has fractured his spine or his neck, there may also be damage to the delicate spinal cord carried by the vertebrae. Unless his life is in danger, it's essential that you don't move your child until an ambulance arrives and that you don't let him move his head. If there is spinal cord injury, your child will experience burning, tingling, or even a loss of sensation in his limbs.

IF YOUR CHILD IS CONSCIOUS

1 **Call an ambulance** as soon as you possibly can or get someone else to do so for you. Comfort and reassure your child and tell him he must try to keep as still as he possibly can.

2 **Put your hands** on either side of his head (don't cover his ears). Steady and support him as you find him – don't move him and don't pull on his neck.

3 **Keep supporting his head** until an ambulance arrives. If possible, get someone else to put some rolled-up blankets or towels around his neck and shoulders to help steady and support him.

4 **If you have help**, add some more blankets and towels at either side of your child's body while you continue to hold his head.

IF YOUR CHILD BECOMES UNCONSCIOUS

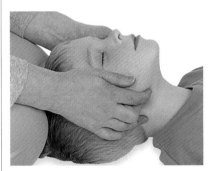

WARNING

- Don't move a child with a spine injury unless his life is in immediate danger
- If he does have to be moved, get as many people to help as you can so that you can lift the child all at once, keeping his body in as straight a line as possible. Don't bend or twist the child's neck or spine.
- Don't tilt his head to open the airway. Lift the jaw instead.

1 **Don't move him**. Stay with him, making sure his body and feet are in a straight line and keeping him as steady as possible.

2 **Open his airway** using the jaw thrust. Kneel behind his head and put your hands on either side of his face. Your fingertips should touch the angles of his jaw. Gently lift his jaw to open the airway.

3 **Check for breathing** and be prepared to give rescue breaths (p.17 baby; p.20 toddler). If he is breathing, support his head until help arrives. If you need to leave your child to call an ambulance, put him in the recovery position before you go (pp.18–19).

EXTREMES OF TEMPERATURE

Extremes of heat and cold affect babies and toddlers more than adults – small bodies cool down and heat up faster than larger ones. And babies aren't able to dress or undress themselves to regulate their temperature.

heat rash

Heat rash is a faint red rash in the areas of the body where there are most sweat glands – the face, neck, shoulders, and skin creases such as the elbows, groin, and behind the knees. Babies often get heat rash because their sweat glands are still developing and not efficient at controlling body temperature.

1 First check your baby's clothing. She may be wearing too many clothes for the air temperature.

2 Undress your baby and bath her in tepid water. Pat her dry to remove most of the moisture, leaving the skin slightly damp. Allow the skin to dry in the air – this will help to cool her down.

3 If the rash hasn't disappeared after 12 hours or your baby has a temperature, call a doctor.

heat exhaustion

Heat exhaustion can develop when a child loses too much body fluid through sweating, or the body becomes overheated in hot humid weather. It isn't usually serious but your child needs cooling as soon as possible.

1 Undress your child and lie her down in a cool, airy room, with a fan if possible.

2 Put something under her head and raise her legs up on some pillows to increase the blood supply to the brain. Let her rest.

3 Tepid sponging will make her feel more comfortable. Also, give her sips of cool salty water – add a teaspoon of salt to a litre of water – or some juice to replace the fluid she has lost.

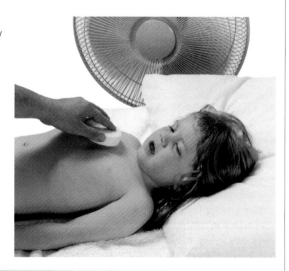

heatstroke

When a baby or toddler is exposed to extreme heat, such as strong sun, the immature temperature control mechanisms and sweat glands may not work properly. Heatstroke can even be fatal and can cause seizures (p.57). If her temperature rises above 40°C (104°F) call an ambulance, and cool her down.

1 First undress your baby and call an ambulance. Bathe her in tepid water. Pat her dry, leaving the skin slightly damp.

2 Allow the skin to dry in the air – this will cool her down. Don't let her get too cool or there's a risk of hypothermia (see below).

3 If she's unconscious, open her airway, check her breathing, and be ready to give rescue breaths (p.17 baby; p.20 toddler).

hypothermia

In this serious condition the body's temperature drops very low. It can be fatal as vital organs such as the heart and liver slow down and stop. A baby can get hypothermia from sleeping in a cold room, prolonged contact with cold water, or from not being properly dressed in cold weather.

WARNING
- Never use a hot-water bottle or other direct heat to treat hypothermia. Warm the child slowly with blankets and clothes.

IN A BABY

1 Call a doctor immediately.

2 Warm your baby gradually in a warm room. Wrap her up and hold her next to your warm body.

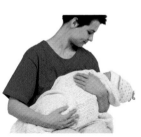

SYMPTOMS
- Shivering
- Cold, pale dry skin
- Listlessness or confusion
- Weak pulse
- Slow, shallow breathing
- Failing consciousness

IN A YOUNG CHILD

1 Give your child a warm, not hot, bath. When her skin colour is normal, dry her and wrap her warmly.

2 Dress her warmly, put a hat on her head and put her to bed in a warm room with a couple of blankets.

3 Give her a warm, not hot, drink and high-energy food. Sit with her until her temperature is normal.

4 If your child's temperature doesn't return to normal, get her to hospital as soon as you can.

WARNING
- If your child loses consciousness, open her airway, and be prepared to begin rescue breathing. Call an ambulance.

POISONING

Symptoms of poisoning include nausea, vomiting, diarrhoea, and unusual sleepiness. Strong poisons can cause loss of consciousness or seizures. If you suspect poisoning, try to identify the poisonous substance.

treating poisoning

Common poisons include household bleach, weedkiller, medicines, and plants such as berries, irises and daffodils, and fungi.

WARNING
- Any young child who has eaten or drunk a potentially poisonous substance should be seen by a doctor.

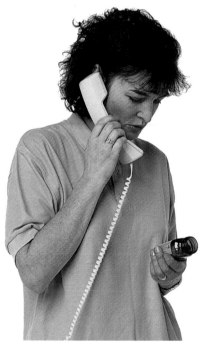

1 **Identify what your child has taken** as quickly as you can.

2 **Call an ambulance**, and tell them as much as possible about what the child has taken and how much (take the container with you to the telephone if necessary). If your child is vomiting you may be asked to keep samples for ambulance personnel.

3 **Monitor your child's vital signs** – level of consciousness, breathing and pulse (p.12) while waiting for help. Depending on what you child has taken there may be additional action to take, see opposite.

4 **If your child loses consciousness**, open his airway, check his breathing and be prepared to give rescue breaths (p.17 baby; p.20 toddler). Stay with him and ask someone to call the ambulance for you. If he has taken a poisonous chemical, protect yourself with a face mask if you need to give rescue breaths.

PREVENTION

- Store medicines in a locked cupboard or on a high shelf. Throw away unused or old medicines.
- Keep disinfectants and bleach locked away in their original containers, preferably with child-resistant tops. When they're in use, keep them out of your child's reach.

- Don't leave alcohol or cigarettes lying around.
- Make sure that any poisonous plants are removed and pull up all types of fungi as soon as they appear.
- Store garden chemicals, such as weedkiller, in a locked shed.

specific types of poisoning

ALCOHOL POISONING

1 Try to keep him awake. Check what he drank and tell the ambulance control.

2 Keep a bowl near him as he's likely to vomit.

3 Keep him warm. Alcohol dilates the blood vessels, and can lead to hypothermia.

4 If your child loses consciousness, open his airways, check his breathing and be ready to give rescue breaths (p.17; p.20).

SYMPTOMS
- Alcohol smell on breath
- Flushed face, sweating
- Nausea and vomiting
- Impaired consciousness: the child may wake up if you rouse him but quickly fall asleep again

SWALLOWED CHEMICALS

1 Wipe any chemicals away from his mouth.

2 Take the container of the chemical to give to the doctor at the hospital.

3 If your child loses consciousness, open his airways, check his breathing and be ready to give rescue breaths (p.17; p.20). Use a face mask over his mouth and nose (baby) or mouth (toddler) to protect yourself from the chemical.

SYMPTOMS
- Pain or burning sensation in gullet
- Burns or blistering around the mouth

PLANT POISONING

1 Check inside his mouth and encourage your child to spit out any bits of leaf or berries still in his mouth.

2 Keep a sample of the plant (leaf or berry) to give to the doctor.

3 Keep a bowl near him as he's likely to vomit

4 Monitor your child's vital signs (p.12) and watch for any changes.

SYMPTOMS
- Abdominal pain
- Nausea and vomiting and later diarrhoea

DRUG POISONING

1 Tell your child to spit out any pills left in his mouth, have a look in his mouth yourself as well and pick out anything you can clearly see. Get your child to hospital as soon as possible. Ingestion of some medications such as paracetamol may result in permanent damage.

2 Monitor your child's vital signs (p.12), looking especially for any deterioration while waiting for help.

SYMPTOMS
- Nausea and vomiting, later diarrhoea
- Abdominal pain
- Drowsiness and possible unconsciousness
- Over-excited, hyperactive behaviour

ILLNESS AND MEDICAL PROBLEMS

Almost every baby and toddler will become ill at some point. Most will suffer from minor ailments such as teething pain or nappy rash. Diarrhoea and vomiting are common signs of a tummy bug, though if either persist you should consult your doctor. Other illnesses covered in this section can be very serious – in particular you should familiarize yourself carefully with the symptoms of meningitis (p.56).

fever

A fever is a temperature of 37.7°C (100°F) or over. An infection is the usual cause, but if your child has a bad headache, check for meningitis (p.56). Always call a doctor if a baby under six months has a fever, or if it is over 40°C (104°F). Babies and toddlers risk febrile seizures (p.57) if their temperature goes too high.

SYMPTOMS

Signs of fever
- Raised temperature
- Child may shiver and look cold and pale

As the fever progresses a child may have:
- Flushed, sweaty skin
- Aching limbs and body
- Headache

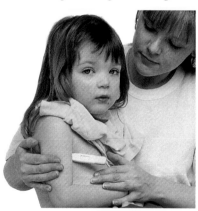

1 **If you think your child** may have a fever, take her temperature (p.13). Note it down and check again 20 minutes later.

3 **Unless your child** is under three months old, you can give the recommended dose of paracetamol syrup. This should help bring down the fever.

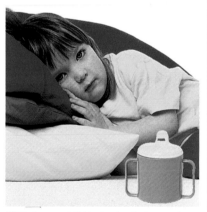

2 **Put your child to bed** or lie her on the sofa. Don't cover her. Give her water or diluted fruit juice to drink.

4 **Undress your child** leaving her skin bare. Don't sponge her with tepid water unless her temperature is exceedingly high or she's having a seizure (p.57). Doctors believe a high temperature is a protective mechanism for killing off viruses and bacteria.

diarrhoea

Diarrhoea (loose watery stools) is always serious in a baby because of the dangers of dehydration. Diarrhoea with vomiting in a toddler is also serious for the same reason, especially if accompanied by fever and sweating.

1 **If your baby is under 12 months** and has had diarrhoea for six hours with other signs of illness, call your doctor immediately.

2 **If your child also has pain** around her navel and to the lower right side of her groin, call the doctor. It might be **appendicitis**.

3 **If your baby has severe abdominal** cramps, vomiting, and blood and mucus in her stools, call your doctor at once. It might be **intussusception** (bowel blockage).

4 **Don't give an older child any food or milk**, but give frequent drinks of rehydration solution, which you can buy as a powder at the chemist.

5 **Check your child's temperature** to see if she has a fever and tell your doctor what the temperature is.

6 **Pay close attention to hygiene,** for instance after changing nappies, to stop infection spreading to the rest of the family

vomiting

Persistent vomiting should always be taken seriously in a baby or young child because of the risk of dehydration.

1 **If your child continues to vomit** over a period of six hours, or has vomiting accompanied by diarrhoea, fever or other symptoms such as earache, call your doctor immediately.

2 **Let your child rest** with a bowl nearby for her to vomit into if necessary.

3 **Give your child small sips** of rehydration solution.

4 **Check her temperature** and keep her cool by sponging with tepid water.

5 **Once the vomiting has passed,** reintroduce solid foods slowly and give only bland foods.

PREVENTING TRAVEL SICKNESS

Some young children suffer from nausea when travelling because the movement upsets the balance organs in the ear. Most children outgrow the problem.

• Don't make a fuss before you travel since this can make your child more nervous and apprehensive.

• Don't let your child travel on an empty or full stomach. Give her a small snack before you leave and don't let her eat lots on the journey.

• Take plenty of drinks with you so your child doesn't become dehydrated.

• Prevent travel sickness by giving your child a travel-sickness medicine beforehand. Several brands are available at chemists.

• Try your child with pressure bands to wear around her wrists. These may work by stimulating acupuncture points.

• If your child suffers from frequent travel sickness, consult your doctor.

meningitis

This is an inflammation of the membranes that cover the brain and spinal cord, caused by a viral or bacterial infection. Viral meningitis is more common and usually not as severe as bacterial meningitis which can be fatal. Both should be treated as an emergency. The sooner treatment is given, the better the chances of recovery.

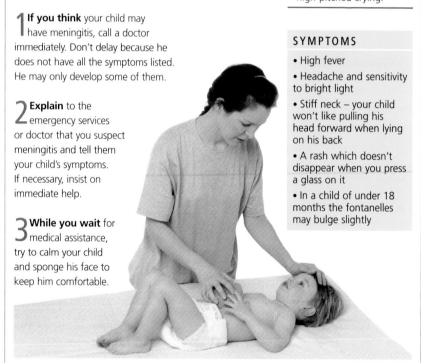

1 **If you think** your child may have meningitis, call a doctor immediately. Don't delay because he does not have all the symptoms listed. He may only develop some of them.

2 **Explain** to the emergency services or doctor that you suspect meningitis and tell them your child's symptoms. If necessary, insist on immediate help.

3 **While you wait** for medical assistance, try to calm your child and sponge his face to keep him comfortable.

WARNING

If you spot any of the symptoms below, call your doctor immediately. A child may also have a fever, drowsiness, and nausea. A baby may be reluctant to feed and have high-pitched crying.

SYMPTOMS

• High fever

• Headache and sensitivity to bright light

• Stiff neck – your child won't like pulling his head forward when lying on his back

• A rash which doesn't disappear when you press a glass on it

• In a child of under 18 months the fontanelles may bulge slightly

HOW TO RECOGNIZE THE MENINGITIS RASH

To check a rash you suspect may be a sign of meningitis, press a clear drinking glass against it. If the rash is still visible through the glass, call the doctor at once.

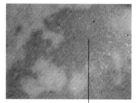

Rash on dark skin

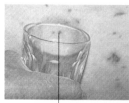

Rash on light skin

seizures

Seizures are also called convulsions or fits. The most common causes of seizures in young children are high fever (known as a febrile seizure), epilepsy, head injury, and poisoning. Seizures usually occur on isolated occasions, but children with epilepsy have repeated attacks.

SYMPTOMS

Febrile seizures
• Child may be flushed and sweaty and have a very hot forehead
• May clench her fists and stiffen and arch her back
• Eyes may roll upwards or be fixed or squinting
• May hold her breath, making face look blue

Epileptic seizures
• Loss of consciousness
• Clenching of teeth
• Stiffness, followed by rhythmic jerking of the limbs
• Involuntary urination
• Frothing of the mouth
• Breathing may stop
• Seizure may be followed by deep sleep

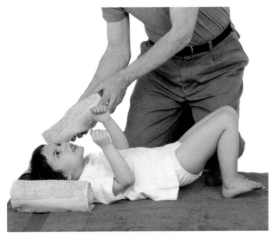

1 If your child is making violent movements, clear away any furniture or objects that she may knock against. Place pillows or other soft padding around your child to protect her from injury.

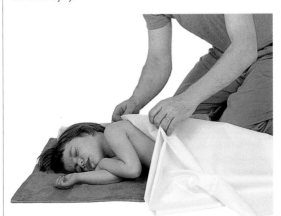

2 Undress your child and make sure she has plenty of fresh air. Do let her become overcooled. If a baby has a seizure and is very hot, sponge her with tepid water.

3 When the seizure is over, place your child in the recovery position (pp.18–19). If her temperature rises, cool her again. If your child has lost consciousness, assess her condition and be prepared to resuscitate (p.18 baby; p.21 toddler). Call an ambulance immediately.

three-month colic

Colic is simply a crying spell, usually in the early evening, when your baby's face becomes very red and she draws both legs up to her stomach as though in pain. The cause is unknown, though colic is so common that doctors regard it as normal. It isn't due to wind, nor is she in pain.

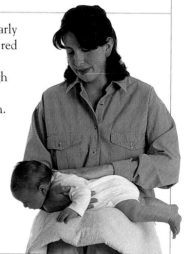

1 Soothe your baby in any way that works at other times – rock her, walk her in a pram, hold her in a sling, or lay her across your lap. A warm bath can also help to soothe a colicky baby.

2 Stay as calm as you can and try not to worry. Each bout can last 1–1½ hours. Colic usually stops by about three months.

teething pain

Teething usually begins at around six or seven months, with most of the first teeth breaking through before 18 months. When a tooth is coming through, you'll feel a hard or sharp lump on your baby's gum and the area will be swollen and red. Symptoms of teething don't include fever, bronchitis, vomiting, diarrhoea, or loss of appetite. These are symptoms of an underlying illness, not of teething.

SYMPTOMS

- Increased saliva and dribbling
- Desire to bite on hard objects
- Irritability and increased clinginess
- Baby finds it hard to sleep
- Swollen red area where new tooth is coming

1 Nurse your baby often to comfort her. Try giving her a chilled (not frozen) teething ring to bite on, or a piece of apple or carrot. Never leave your baby with a piece of food in case she chokes.

2 Rub the swollen gum with your finger to soothe it. Try to avoid teething jellies that contain local anaesthetics as these have only a temporary effect and can sometimes cause an allergy. Only use pain relief on your doctor's advice.

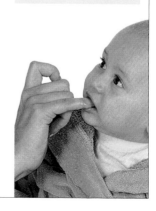

3 If your child refuses food, encourage her to eat by offering cold, smooth foods such as yogurt, ice cream, or jelly. These will soothe her sore gums.

nappy rash

Nappy rash is a skin condition that affects the area covered by a baby's nappy. A common cause is not changing the nappy often enough so the bacteria in the stools act on urine and release irritating ammonia.

1 **If you notice any redness** on your baby's bottom, wash her bottom with warm water and dry well. Apply thick barrier cream to prevent her urine from irritating her skin.

2 **Change nappies and wash** your baby's bottom frequently, at least every 2 to 3 hours and after a bowel motion. Leave her nappy off as often as possible.

3 **Don't use talcum powder** around your baby's genitals as this cakes when wet and may irritate the skin.

4 **Check the inside** of your baby's mouth. If you notice white patches, try to wipe them off with a clean handkerchief. If they leave raw, red patches, your baby may have oral thrush, which can cause nappy rash.

5 **Check with your doctor** if your baby has oral thrush or if her nappy rash does not clear up in two or three days.

SYMPTOMS

- Redness over the nappy area
- Redness that starts around the genitals and is accompanied by a strong smell of ammonia
- Tight, papery skin with inflamed spots that have pus-filled centres.
- Redness that starts around the anus and moves over the buttocks and on to the thighs

ear pain

Earache may have a number of causes, the most common of which is infection of the middle ear. Pain in the ear may also be caused by toothache, tonsillitis or mumps, or by a foreign object in the external canal of the ear (p.44).

1 **Call your doctor** immediately if your child is too young to tell you she's in pain, but is crying, generally off-colour and pulling or rubbing at one of her ears. She might need antibiotics.

2 **Take your child's** temperature in case she has a fever and check for discharge from the ear.

3 **Check with your doctor** immediately if there's a fever and/or discharge.

4 **Make your child** comfortable. Place a hot-water bottle, covered by a towel, next to your child's ear to relieve the pain.

5 **If the pain** doesn't subside, call your doctor.

SYMPTOMS

- Pain around the ear
- Fever of over 38°C (100.4°F)
- Discharge of pus from the ear
- Deafness
- Inflammation of the tonsils
- Pain when the ear is touched
- Swollen glands
- Young child may rub and pull at the ear

SAFETY IN AND AROUND THE HOME

Most accidents to young children happen at home, and many household items are dangerous to children. Make your home and garden "childproof" before your baby learns to crawl or move around – don't wait until she has nearly fallen down the stairs or grabbed a trailing flex before you take action.

general safety rules

Take a good look around your home and check for the following dangers. Make your house as safe as it can be.

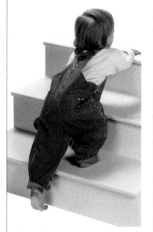

Fit safety gates to all staircases so your child cannot climb them alone.

- **Avoid trailing flexes**, loose carpets, and rugs
- **Keep all electric plug sockets covered** with plastic covers or put heavy furniture in front of them
- **Fit locks to all windows**
- **Fit childproof locks to cupboards and drawers**
- **Make sure that from an early age** your child knows that hot things such as fires and ovens are dangerous and that she should not go near them
- **Keep matches and lighters out of reach** and fit a smoke alarm on every floor of your home
- **Fit safety gates to the top and bottom of your stairs.** Gates at the top of the stairs should open onto the landing and should not have horizontal bars that your baby could climb
- **Keep all medicines, cleaning materials, and poisonous substances** well out of reach in a lockable cupboard. Even vitamin pills are dangerous. Never tell your child that medicines are special sweeties
- **Buy medicines and poisonous substances** with child-resistant tops whenever possible and always keep them in their original containers
- **Don't leave sharp, heavy or hot objects on low tables** or in your baby's reach
- **Fit guards to all fires and to the cooker.** Always point saucepan handles towards the back of the hob
- **Fit special protective edges** on sharp-cornered furniture or door handles
- **Remove glass-topped items** or fit them with safety film
- **Keep the lavatory lid closed**
- **Avoid poisonous houseplants**
- **Stop using tablecloths.** Your child could pull it – and anything on the cloth – on top of herself

safety at bathtime

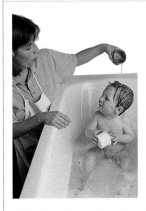

- **When preparing your child's bath**, add hot water to cold, never the other way round
- **Use non-slip mats in the bath**
- **Always check the temperature** of the water before putting your child in. Even older babies need the water considerably cooler than most adults
- **Turn off the taps tightly** before putting your child in the bath and cover the taps with a flannel so she doesn't scald or hurt herself
- **Don't let your baby stand** or jump in the water unsupported
- **Never leave your baby alone** in a bath

safety at bedtime

- **Never leave your baby** with the cot side down
- **Never leave your baby** alone on the changing table, even for a second
- **Don't use a pillow** in your baby's cot until she is one year old
- **Don't leave gas or electric fires** on in a baby's room when she is on her own

Put your baby with her feet at the foot of the cot to stop her slipping under the covers.

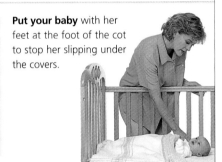

safety outside

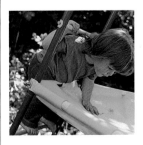

- **Remove any poisonous plants** and pull up any fungi
- **Store garden tools** and chemicals in a locked shed
- **Check safety** of any play equipment regularly
- **Put climbing toys on grass**, not on paved areas
- **Make sure your child cannot run out of the garden** into the road. Fit child-resistant locks to gates
- **Fence off and cover ponds and swimming pools**
- **Don't allow pets to defecate** in the garden
- **Cover sandpits** to prevent fouling by animals

index

emergency numbers

In the event of an emergency call 999 and ask for the police, ambulance or fire brigade.

For other health information in England and Wales call NHS Direct on 0845 4647.
In Scotland for referrals call the NHS Helpline on 0800 224488.

It's worth making a note here of your doctor's telephone number and the number of your local accident and emergency department.

Doctor:

....

Local accident and emergency department:

....

first aid courses

St. John Ambulance, St. Andrew Ambulance Association (in Scotland), and the British Red Cross all run First Aid courses. For more information contact the relevant organization.

St. John Ambulance:
call 08700 10 49 50
or visit www.sja.org.uk

St. Andrew Ambulance Association (in Scotland):
call 0141 332 4031
or visit www.firstaid.org.uk

British Red Cross:
contact your local British Red Cross office or visit www.redcross.org.uk

acknowledgments

picture credits
Picture research: Anna Bedewell
Picture librarians: Hayley Smith and Romaine Werblow
The publisher would like to thank the following for their kind permission to reproduce their photographs:
(Abbreviations key: b=bottom, r=right, c=centre)

56: Meningitis Research Foundation (bc, br)

All other pictures © Dorling Kindersley.
For further information see **www.dkimages.com**